Maria Theiopoulou

# Pillow Yoga

To all my lazy friends...

*Whenever I feel the need to exercise,*
*I lie down until it goes away.*
**Paul Terry**
*(the animator of Mighty Mouse)*

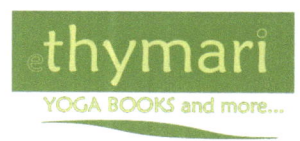

easy...relaxing...effective

# Pillow Yoga

enjoyable...therapeutic

**a guide for a gentle approach of yoga
with the use of simple sofa pillows**

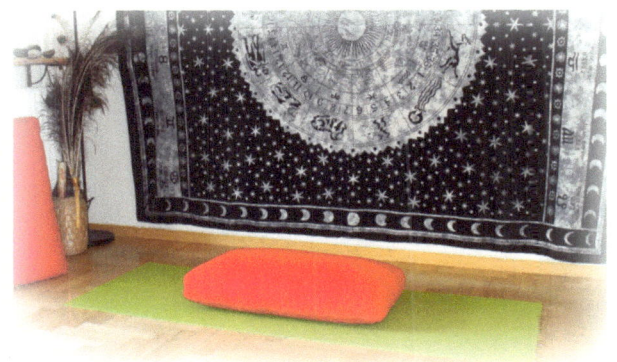

Maria Theiopoulou

**Photos by Julian Venter**

# Pillow Yoga

**Who is it for**

Everybody who likes it and needs it, no matter what age or level of fitness.

**When to practice**

Whenever you feel like stretching and relaxing. When experiencing headaches, sinus blockages, asthma attacks, stomach aches, indigestion, menstrual pains, fatigue or anxiety strikes.

**Where to practice**

Wherever you can find sofa pillows and peace. In your house, yoga studio, gym, hotel room, private office.

**How to practice**

Using sofa pillows and a yoga mat on the floor. Do not use bed pillows, because they are too small, soft and unstable. Also do not practice in bed. You need a hard surface to straighten your spine correctly.

**Why practice it**

To enjoy yoga in an easy and comfortable way. To restore your body alignment. To stretch into positions that feel difficult otherwise. To prepare for more advanced training.

# The benefits

## Support

You can relax deeply into the poses. The support provided by the pillows cultivates a sense of safety in the body and the mind. The softness of the pillow also enhances the feeling of surrender on a psychological level.

## Progress

By letting your body get used to the poses in an easy way, you are building the trust it needs to expand more. This way you make effortless and fast progress.

## Enjoyment

It really feels so pleasant, that there is not one moment of discomfort. The only difficulty is convincing yourself not to spend all day on the pillows.

## Therapy

By aligning and opening the body effortlessly, recovery and possibly cure become reality. This easy, relaxing practice calms the mind and frees blocked emotions, thus helping to resolve psychological problems.

............................ Tip ............................

Make your pillows even more pleasant with a few drops of essential oil. Choose the essence you prefer each time and enjoy a combination of soft yoga and aromatherapy. *Suggestions*: **Lavender** for deep relaxing, **Neroli** for relieving headache and anxiety, **Lemon** for coolness and vitality, **Geranium** for clear mind and concentration, **Bergamot** for increasing self confidence, **Cedar** or **Patchouli** for feelings of warmth and safety, **Jasmine** or **Ylang ylang** for sensuality.

# Easy Seat

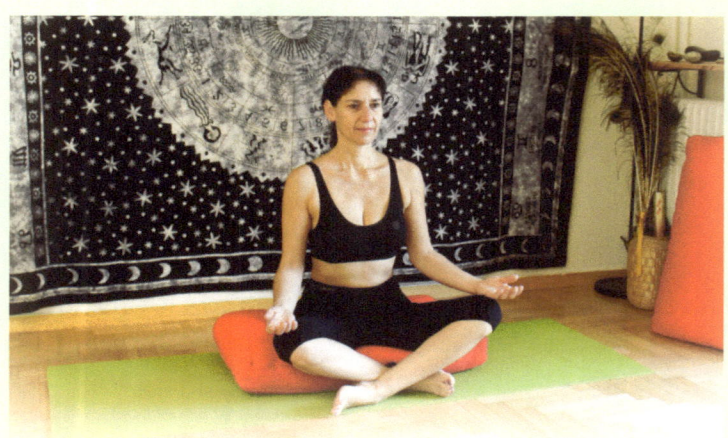

Sit in the crossed legged position with the pelvis on the pillow and the feet on the floor. Gently lift your back and neck, as if you are being pulled up from the top of the head. Breathe deeply and evenly. If you can't, just observe your breathing as it is, without judgment or effort to change it. This will allow it to naturally become deep and even.

Hold the spine elongated and centered, using your abdominals and upper back muscles. Look straight ahead, in order to secure the right position for the neck. You can change the legs and cross them the other way around whenever you feel like it.

Now you can close the eyes. Relax the arms and the hands. Imagine them as water streaming down, from the shoulders to the finger tips. Imagine your pelvis as a solid rock rooted deeply in the earth, the torso as a trunk of a tree that keeps growing upwards and the head as the flower that opens towards the sun.

# Saint

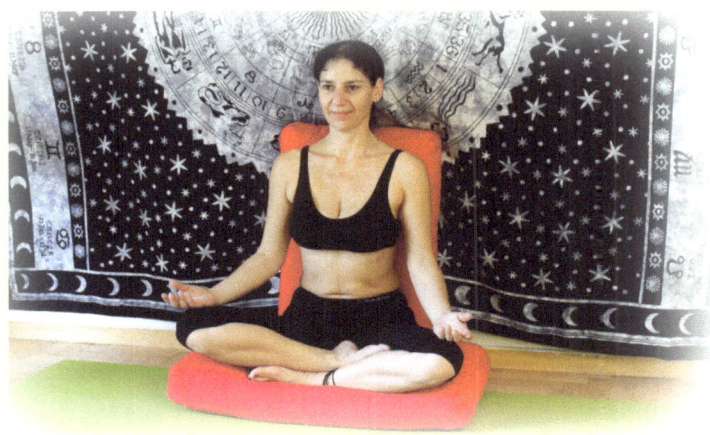

Struggling to sit with your back straight? Lean on the wall and sit in the pose of the Saint. Place one foot in front of the other. You can also use one more pillow to support your back. Use the abdominals to lift the torso. Once they become strong enough, you won't need the wall anymore.

Change the feet whenever you feel like it. You can also close your eyes and meditate.

## Benefits

Both poses provide flexibility to the knees and ankles, relieve from pain of menstruation, ease breathing and develop calmness and concentration. They are perfect for meditation and the ancient yoga scriptures say that they purify the energy channels and cure all diseases.

# Spinal Twists

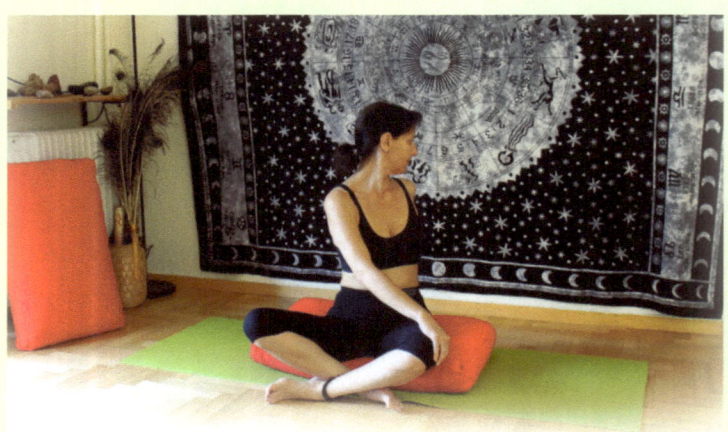

In the Easy Seat, hold the knee with the opposite hand and the pillow from behind with the other. Lengthen the spine and neck, keep the torso vertically centered and turn with every exhalation. Repeat on the other side.

You can do continuous twists or stay for five to ten breaths in each side. Exhale generously, pulling the side of the belly in until all the air is out. Change the leg crossing, if you need to, and repeat on both sides.

## Benefits

The Spinal Twists give elasticity to the spine and can help cure scoliosis, if you stay longer in the affected side. Also they detoxify the intestines, relieve from indigestion and dissolve belly fat. The turning of the chest opens the lungs and eases breathing, while the muscles of the back become longer and stronger.

# Side Stretches

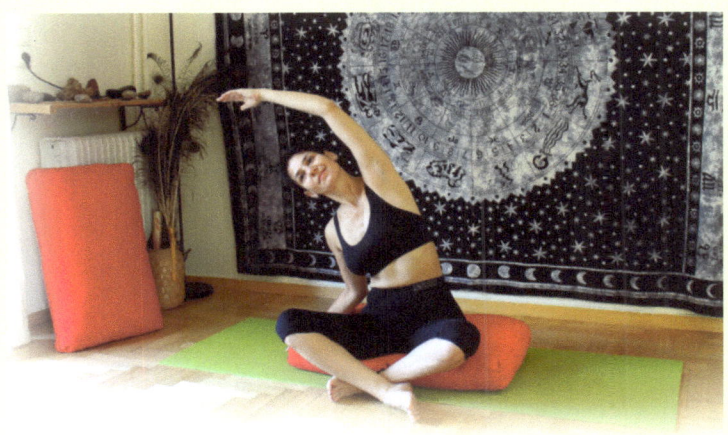

Hold the side of the pillow, stretch your arm and torso and lengthen sideways as far as you can, holding both sides of the pelvis down. Elongate the neck and let it follow the spine. Imagine your upper body as a young tree, gracefully leaning with the wind. Repeat on the other side.

If you suffer from arthritis or you just don't feel comfortable lifting your arm high, just place the palm behind the head, holding the elbow as open as you can.

## Benefits

While maintaining all the benefits of the Spinal Twists, the Side Stretches open and elongate the rib cage, in a move that we almost never do in everyday life. The torso becomes stronger and more flexible and the internal organs get a detoxifying massage.

# Seated Backward Bend

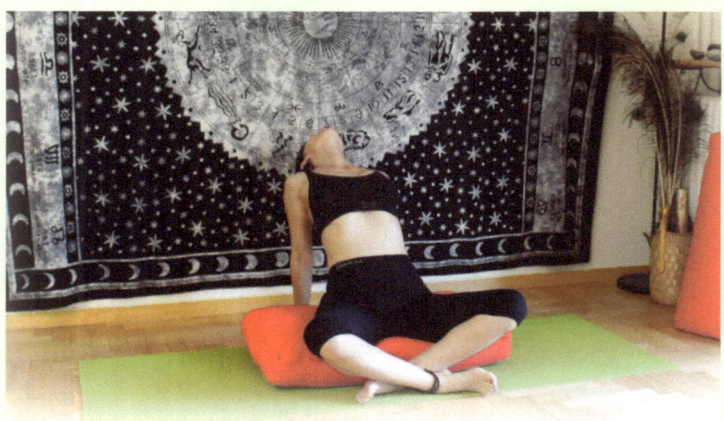

Place the palms on the floor behind the pillow, with the fingers pointed forwards. Lift the chest and look up. Take the opportunity to breathe deeply, now that the lungs are wide open. Stay as long as you feel comfortable.

Accept guidance and help from the sky. New ideas might come to you and old emotional blockages could be released.

To come back, first bring the head forward and then the torso and hands. You can change the legs and repeat.

## Benefits

It relieves and can gradually cure heart and breathing problems, cultivates optimism and openness towards life. Very effective against depression and phobias. It also strengthens the arms and hands and burns belly fat, preventing diabetes.

# Seated Forward Bend

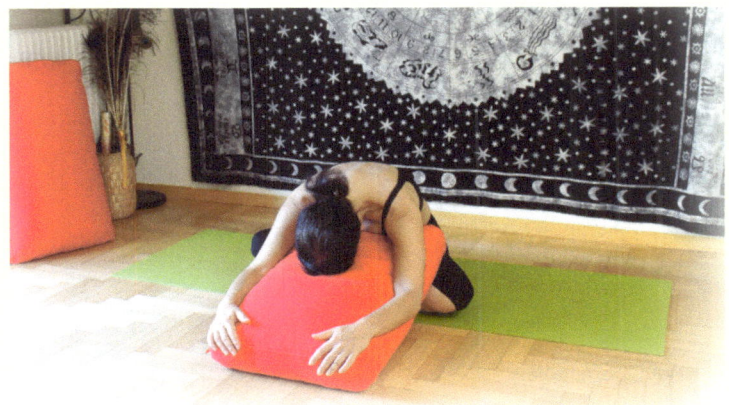

Place the pillow on the feet. You may prefer to cross the feet in the Saint pose first, otherwise it can be hard on the ankles. Leave the pelvis heavy and steady on the floor and relax the chest, hands and forehead on the pillow.

Stay and breath, emphasizing on the exhalations. Every now and then stretch your torso further and let it fall on the pillow again. Let your neck lengthen by keeping the shoulders away from the ears. Feel the support and comfort of the earth and let all your worries melt away.

## Benefits

The Seated Forward Bend releases blockages in the spine and pelvis, while the opening of the legs benefits the reproductive system. Psychologically it gives a sense of safety and acceptance, very effective for alleviating insecurity, indecision and unexpressed grief.

# Diamond

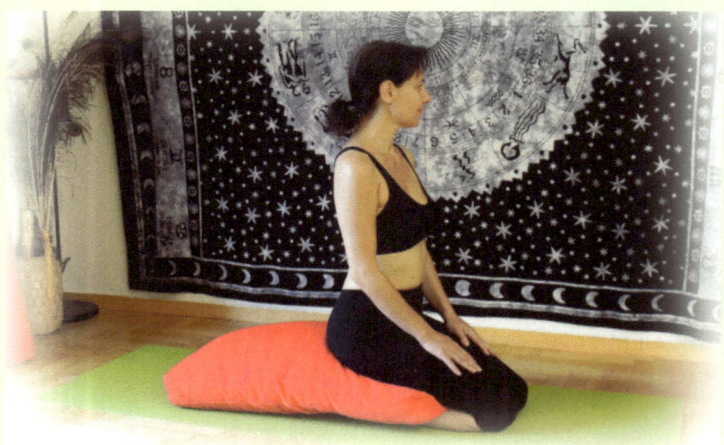

Place the pillow between the pelvis and the heels and sit on it with all your weight. If the front of the feet hurt, take a break and try it again. You can also put a folded blanket underneath to make it easier.

Let your palms rest on the thighs. Hold the back straight and the neck long, looking straight ahead. Loosen the shoulders and arms. Let your breathing become deep, even and relaxed.

The Diamond is an ideal pose for neck and shoulder exercises. Gently let the head fall back and forth, then turn and lean left and right (see next page). Make slow circles with your head, keeping the eyes closed to avoid dizziness. If you suffer from neck pain, make sure you move your head softly and carefully and do the neck exercises every day. Next you can roll your shoulders backwards and forwards.

It is also a very good position for utilizing yogic belly breath-

# Neck exercises

Head backwards

Head forwards

Head turning right and left

Head leaning right and left

ing. When inhaling, send the air as low into your abdominal region as you can, letting the belly expand. When exhaling, blow all the air out and gently push the belly inwards. This way you can cleanse the lungs, strengthen the heart and the abdominals and relaxes your nervous system.

## Benefits

The Diamond pose gives flexibility to the knees and relaxes the feet after prolonged standing, therapeutic for varicose veins. It stimulates the digestive system and is ideal for healing dyspepsia, gastritis and ulcers. It helps breathing and concentration, calms the mind and can be used as a meditation posture. It is the only yoga pose that is recommended to be performed after a meal.

The neck exercises release tension in the head and correct the neck position. The shoulder's circular movements dissolve headaches and relieve the symptoms of arthritis.

# Stretching the Arms Behind

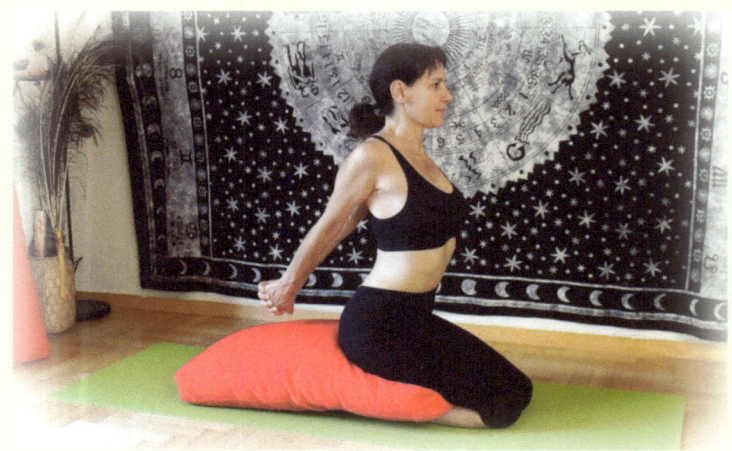

Interlace your fingers behind the lower back. If you can, press the palms together. Stretch the arms down and backward, holding the shoulders down and the neck long and soft. Keep lifting up the stomach and look straight ahead. Release the hands and repeat, as many times as you feel like.

Try to interlace the fingers differently every time, by changing the thumbs. It might feel awkward in the beginning, but it is a very good and simple method for dissolving mental obsessions, by experiencing an alternative way to do things.

Breathe deeply in this position, as the lungs are wide open.

·························· **Tip** ·······················

If you are experiencing severe neck or lower back pain, take it easy or avoid it until you feel better.

# Stretching the Arms Up

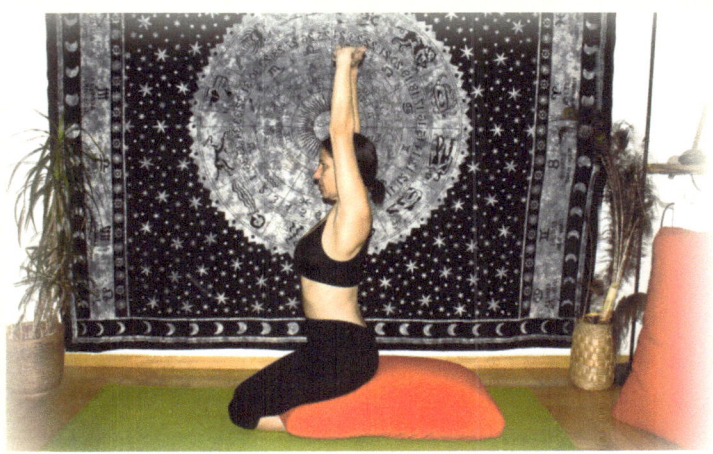

Interlace your fingers and stretch the arms up, elbows next to the ears, if you can. Keep the shoulders down and the neck long and soft, even if you have to bend your arms to do so. Look straight ahead.

You can also move the arms, bringing the elbows behind the ears and back. If you are suffering from arthritis, take it easy and do what you can, but stick with this exercise. With time and patience it will help you very much to regain your shoulders' mobility.

## Benefits

Maintaining all the benefits of the basic Diamond pose, these stretches strengthen the hands, arms, back and neck, align the spine and open the lungs.

# Embryo

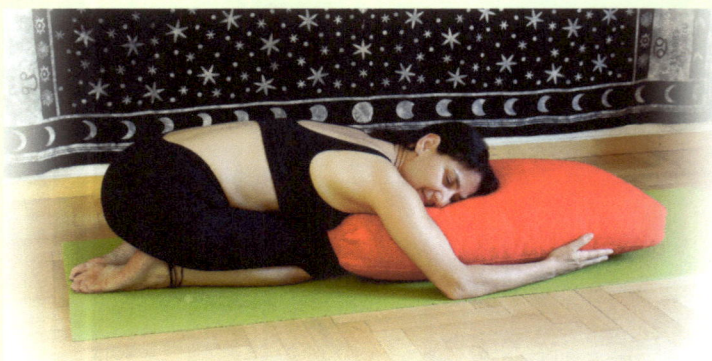

Sit steadily on your heels and place the pillow in front of your knees. Lean forward, hug the pillow and rest on a cheek. Stop all effort and surrender to gravity. Stay as long as you want and change cheeks every now and then. Exhale completely, setting all your worries free. The earth will happily receive them and recycle them into positive energy.

To come back push the pelvis on the heels and let the spine unfold naturally, one vertebra at a time, raising the head last.

## Benefits

The Embryo pose lengthens the spine and relieves backache and neck stiffness, while stretching and relaxing the leg muscles. It stimulates the digestive and reproductive systems and regulates the thyroid function. Beneficial to eyesight, hearing, teeth and hair, it also calms the nerves, bringing us in touch with our inner world. The Embryo on the pillow gives you a perfect sense of comfort and safety. Here you can release all tension under the protection of mother earth and feel like a baby again.

# Tiger Stretch

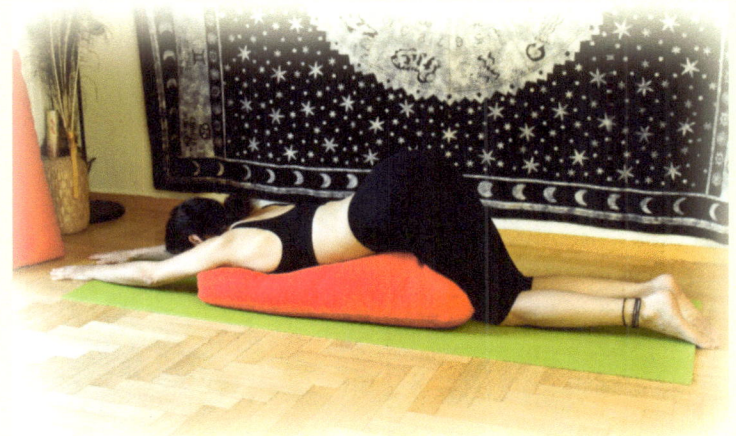

Lift the pelvis and walk your hands forward, letting the chest rest on the pillow. Place your chin over the front side of the pillow. Find your most comfortable position and surrender, allowing the spine to relax and stretch.

To come back, bring the hands closer and support the upper body, until the pelvis can safely sit on the heels.

## Benefits

The Tiger Stretch gives flexibility to the back and lower back and relief from sciatica. It loosens up the legs and stretches the abdominals. It promotes digestion, stimulates blood circulation and restores vitality to the reproductive system. It is also a good warm-up for the spine and pelvis for more challenging exercises.

# Cat

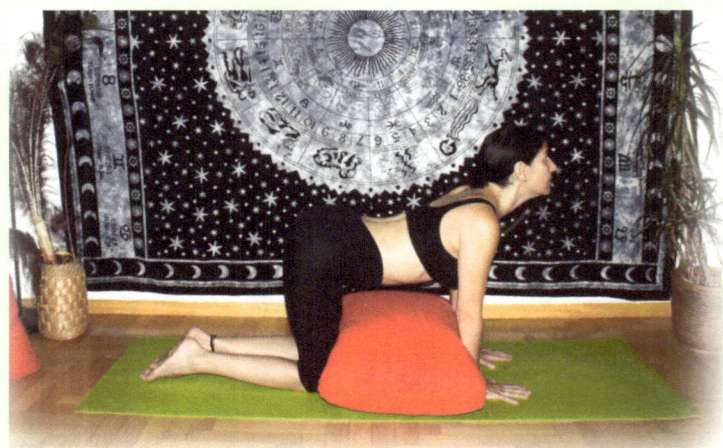

Place the palms firmly on the ground and lift your pelvis, torso and head. Arch as much as you can, while maintaining the elasticity of the spine.

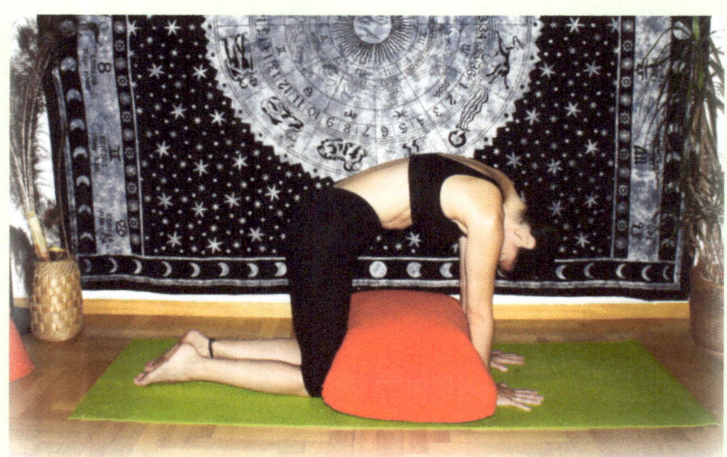

Round the back, sucking the belly and stomach in, keep the shoulders open and the neck free and long.

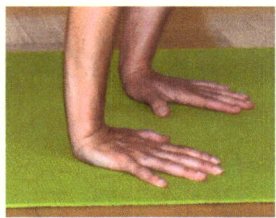

The hands in the Cat position must be firmly placed on the floor, like stickers, with the whole palm and all the fingers pressing down steadily. The same applies for the Dog (p.24).

The Cat is one of the basic and most important yoga exercises. It aligns, elongates and unblocks the spine, thus resolving issues of the neck, shoulders, back and lower back. At the same time it strengthens the hands, arms, legs and feet and benefits greatly the reproductive system, preventing and relieving menstrual pains and increasing fertility.

The pillow gives you the right distance between the hands and the knees, which is vital for the correct performance of the exercise. Place your arms vertically to the floor and make sure that your knees are slightly open, parallel and in line with the hands. If the mat feels too hard, place a folded blanket under the knees.

## Benefits

The Cat exercise gives flexibility to the spine and relieves back and lower back pain. It facilitates breathing and strengthens the wrists. It is particularly beneficial during menstruation, as it helps the blood flow, thus eases pain. It is also a good warm-up of the spine and pelvis for more challenging postures, like the Dog and the Dolphin.

# Rabbit

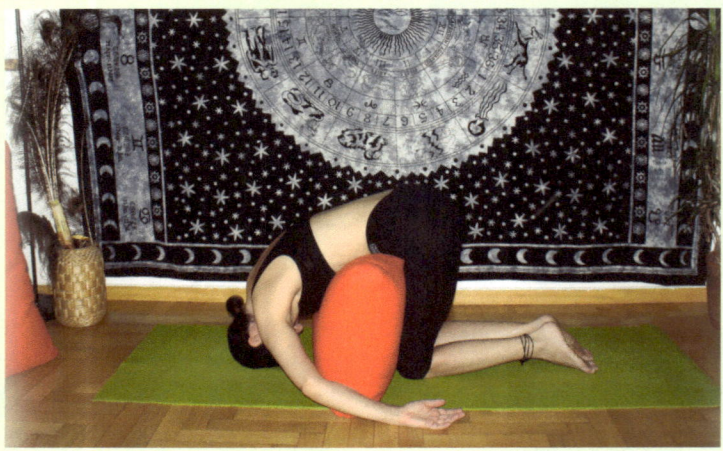

Sit on your knees and place the pillow on the front of the thighs. With the help of your hands carefully lean over the pillow, until the top of the head touches the floor. Hold your legs and feet strong, your abdominals energized and let the arms rest next to the knees, the elbows loose. Keep your neck long, by not putting all your weight on the head.

When you are ready to come up, slowly bring the pelvis back on the heels and let your spine follow, one vertebra at a time.

## Benefits

The Rabbit regulates the thyroid, improves eyesight and hearing and strengthens the hair. It relieves asthma and sinusitis, calms the mind, stimulates the digestive and reproductive systems and relaxes the body after standing poses and backbends. The pillow holds the belly in and allows the shoulders to loosen up completely.

# Camel

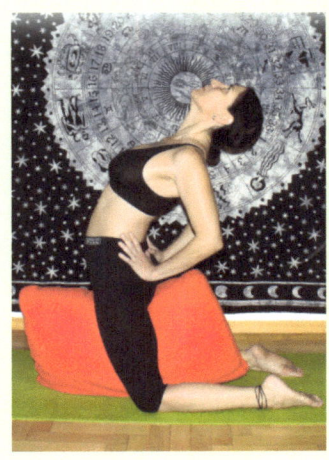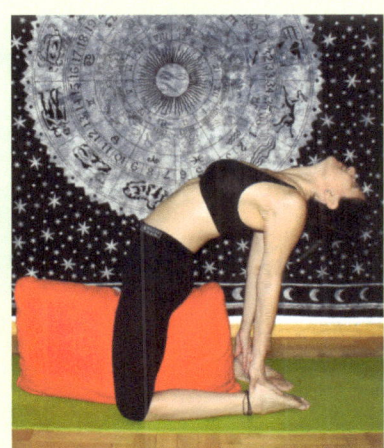

Hold the pillow firmly between your knees and press the feet onto the floor. Support the pelvis with the hands and elongate the torso as much as you can, arching backwards. You can stay here and keep opening the chest. If your lower back is up for it, you can arch all the way until your hands touch your heels. Let the head fall back freely and push the pelvis as far forward as possible. To come up, put the hands on the lower back, bring the head back first and then the torso. Be careful and aware, as this is an intense stretch and needs to be performed with caution and safety.

## Benefits

The Camel pose corrects the curvature of the spine, lengthens the front leg muscles, removes tension from the stomach and stimulates the immune and reproductive systems. It regulates the thyroid, facilitates breathing and, most important, opens the heart. The pillow in this pose helps the knees to remain parallel, which is essential for the protection of the spine.

# Hero

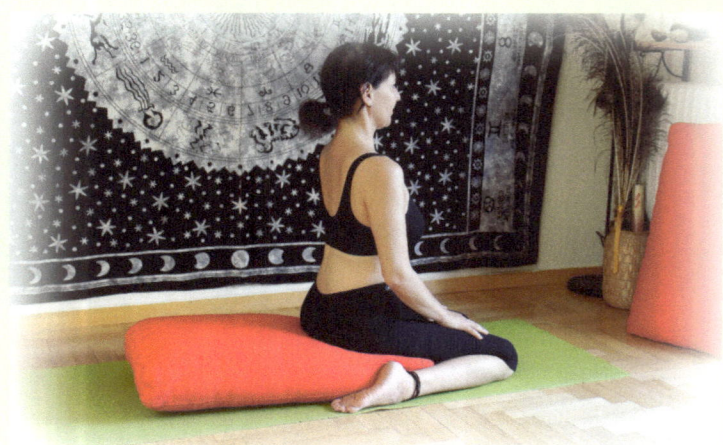

Open the knees and place the pillow between the legs. Let the pelvis sit steadily and hold the torso and neck long and the shoulders relaxed. Don't put any pressure on the knees, only relax the front leg muscles and let them elongate, with the help of the exhalations.

If the knees or the metatarsal bones hurt, don't stay long. This pose requires a gentle and patient approach. In time it will reward you with flexible legs and joints.

## Benefits

The Hero gives all the benefits of the Diamond pose, with the added advantage of a feeling of grounding, as the pelvis sits closer to the floor. The pillow gives you the option of a gentle approach, before you can try the actual position, with the pelvic floor touching the ground directly and the knees folding even more.

# Supine Hero

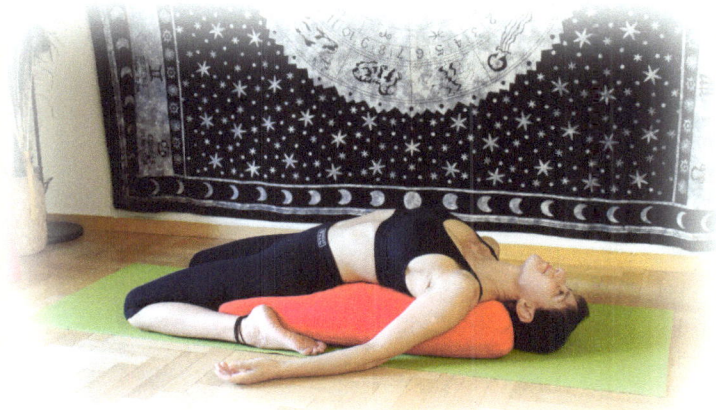

From the Hero pose let the back spread evenly on the pillow. Use your hands for support and let them go only when you are lying on the pillow completely comfortably, with the spine long and the head relaxing back on the floor.

Come up slowly by pushing the elbows down while holding the heels. Bring the head back first, then the torso. Don't move the lower back towards the left or right.

## Benefits

The Supine Hero stretches the abdominal organs, the legs and the spine and opens the chest. It is very effective against dyspepsia, spinal curvature, asthma, depression, phobias and low self esteem. The inclined position of the head benefits the brain, the eyes and the facial skin and contributes to the prevention and reduction of wrinkles.

# Downward Facing Dog

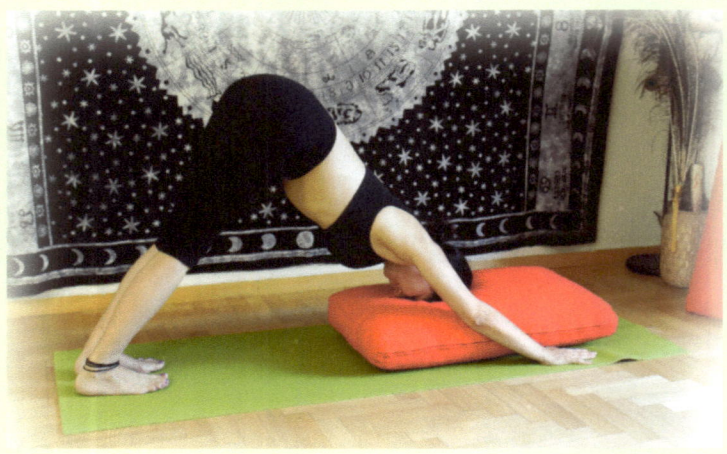

From the Embryo position (p.16) place the palms firmly on the floor, push them down strongly and lift the pelvis. Let the forehead rest on the pillow, while straightening the legs as much as you can. You can walk on the spot, bending one knee after the other, to train the legs for the final position. The heels will probably not touch the floor in the beginning, but this will come with time and practice.

## Benefits

The Downward Facing Dog lengthens the back of the legs, thus detoxifies the entire body. It strengthens the arms and relieves arthritis, stimulates and rejuvenates the spine and corrects the spinal curvature. It cures shortness of breath, headaches and insomnia, relieves tension in the neck and relaxes the heart. It alleviates symptoms of menstrual cramps and menopause, calms the mind, improves memory and restores a positive outlook on life in cases of depression. It compensates fatigue from standing positions and gives energy to the body.

# Dolphin

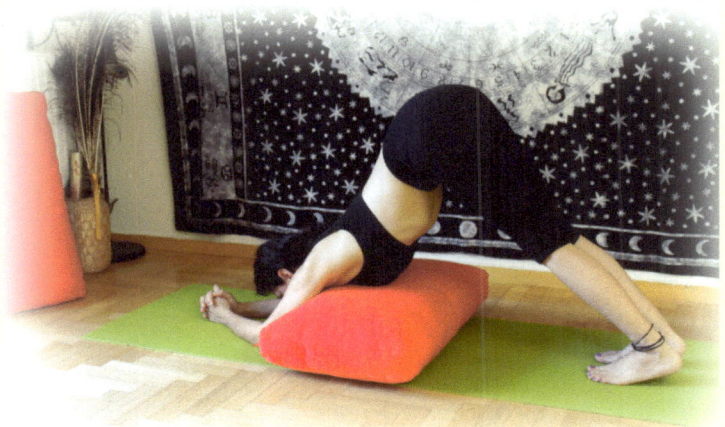

From the Cat pose, place the elbows shoulder distance to each other in front of the pillow and interlace the fingers. Lift the pelvis and straighten the legs. The weight is on the forearms, so you don't need to squeeze the fingers or constrain the shoulders. On the contrary, the neck should be loose and free to move back and forth.

If all this is too much, put the tip of the head on the floor for extra support and walk the legs on the spot to release some of the tension.

## Benefits

The Dolphin has similar benefits to the Dog, but it is more demanding and should be performed carefully. It particularly strengthens the abdominals, the back and the shoulders and allows the chest and pelvis to open up more.

# Pigeon

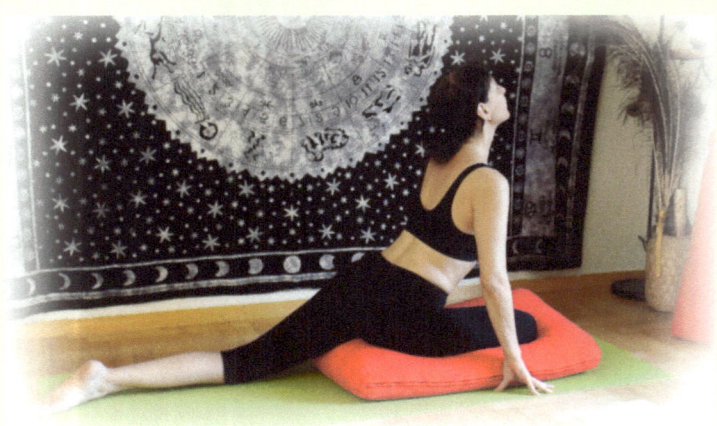

From the Dog pose lift one leg, bend the knee and bring it forwards, placing it on the pillow. Try to keep the pelvis facing forward and let the torso extend upwards, with the top of the head leading. Support yourself with your hands on the finger tips. Press the back foot on the floor, keep the shoulders back, open the chest as much as you can and breathe deeply.

Come back to the Dog by pressing the palms down on the floor and taking the leg back. Repeat with the other leg and hold for the same amount of breaths. The pillow makes the pose easier and prepares you for the final pose, where the pelvic floor touches the ground.

· · · · · · · · · · · · · · · · · · · · · · · **Tip** · · · · · · · · · · · · · · · · · · · · · · ·

If you are experiencing severe back or lower back pain, take it easy or avoid it completely for now.

# Sleeping Pigeon

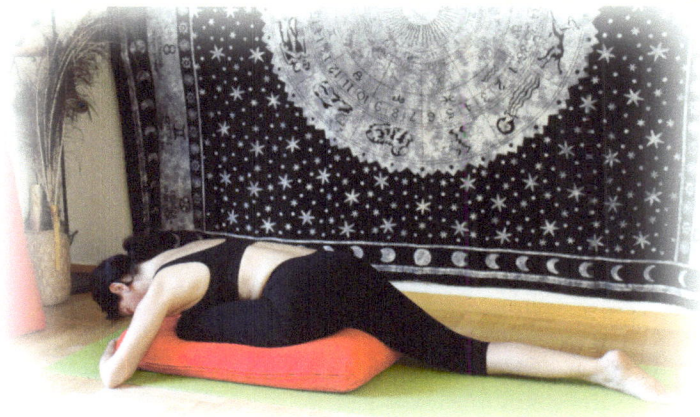

In the Pigeon pose extend the torso forwards and let it fall. Hug the pillow and rest the forehead. Use your exhalations to help the body relax and surrender to gravity.

Come back to the Dog, holding your palms firmly on the floor, and do the other side or do both the Pigeon and the Sleeping Pigeon as a sequence and then repeat with the other leg. Keep your pelvis parallel at all times.

## Benefits

The Pigeon increases the flexibility of the pelvis and spine, lengthens the legs and facilitates breathing. It benefits the reproductive and digestive systems. The Sleeping Pigeon relaxes the back and gives an additional feeling of safety and relief.

# Runner

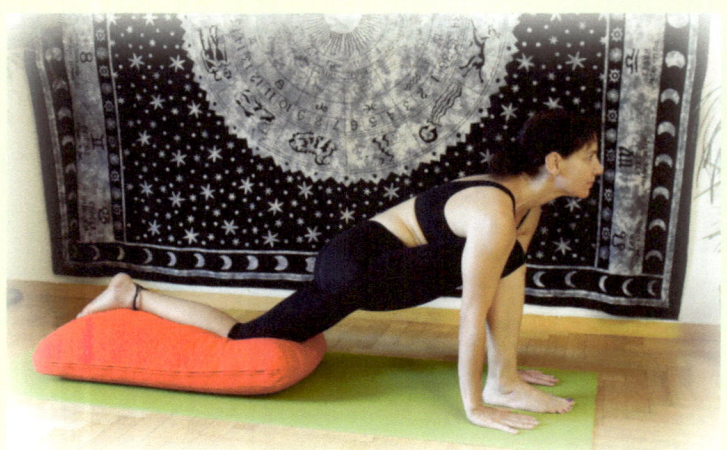

Place one knee on the pillow and the sole of the other foot in front, at a distance of more or less another pillow. Place the hands next to the front foot, extend the torso and neck and look forwards, like a runner about to start a race. Stay for a few breaths and constantly push the pelvis forwards.

Gently come back and repeat with the other leg or proceed to the New Moon pose (next page) and then change side.

## Benefits

The Runner lengthens the legs and corrects the curvature of the spine. It stimulates the immune, digestive and reproductive systems and gives vitality, offsetting the damages caused by the stagnation of a sedentary lifestyle.

# New Moon

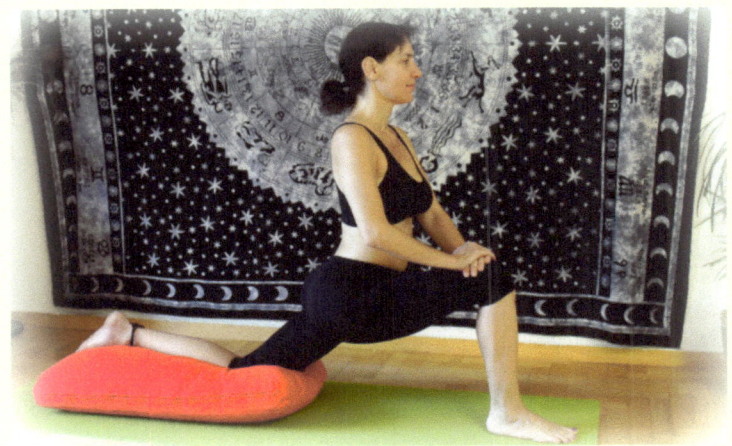

From the Runner press your front foot firmly on the floor and place your hands on the knee. Do not let your knee go over your toes. Engage the abdominals to help your balance and stability. Lengthen the torso and push the pelvis forwards, while looking straight ahead. Relax the shoulders and breathe calmly and deeply.

Repeat on the other side and hold for an equal amount of breaths.

## Benefits

The New Moon maintains all the benefits of the Runner, adding the opportunity to open the chest more, facilitating breathing. It can work miracles for the menstrual cycle, as it opens the channels of the reproductive system, treating menstruation problems and increasing fertility.

# Standing Forward Bend

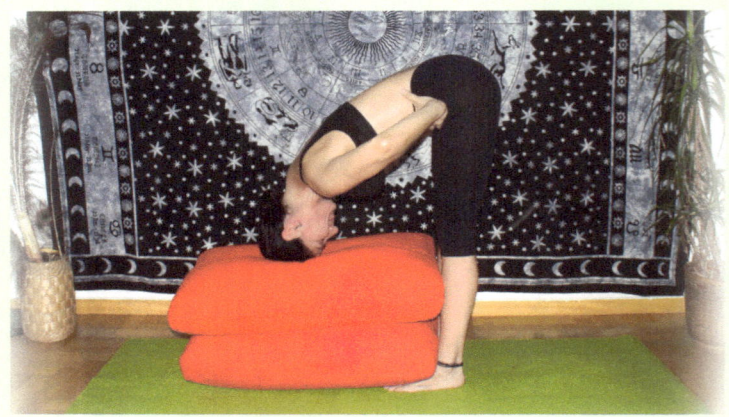

Place two pillows on your feet and lean forwards, until the head touches and rests on the pillows. Place your hands on the waist and pull the belly in on every exhalation. Bring your body weight onto the front of your feet and equalize the weight on either side of each foot.

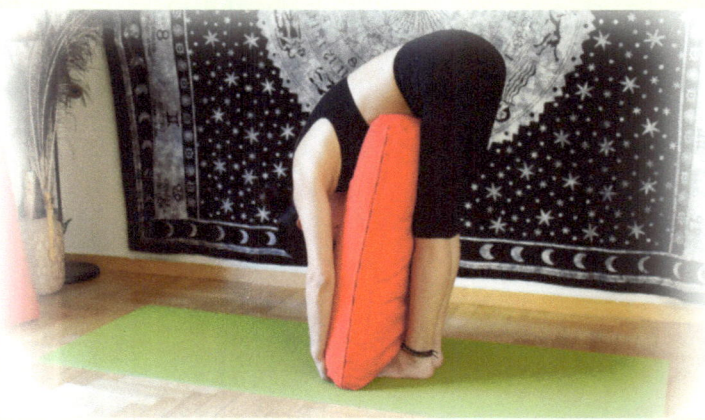

Place one pillow on the feet, so that it touches the front of legs. Draw the belly in and lean over, letting your torso fall freely towards the floor.

For all variations lift the pelvis, keep the legs strong and relax the upper body. Straighten the legs as much as you can. To come up round the back, bend the legs and let the spine unfold gently, one vertebra at a time, the neck and head last.

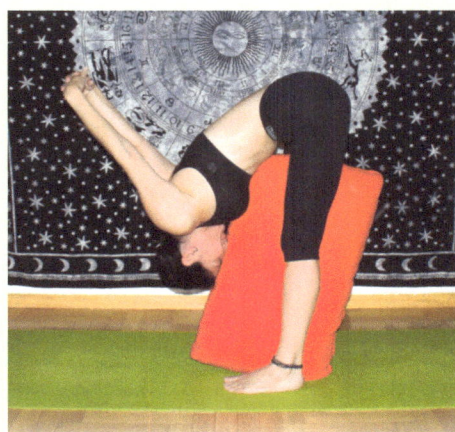
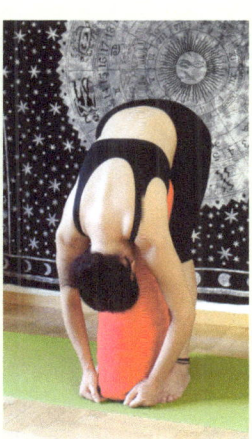

Hold the pillow between your knees and benc. Make the spine long and take the belly in. You can also interlace the fingers behind the back and give it a good, intensive stretch down by straightening the arms and bringing them forwards. Release the arms carefully, keeping the shoulders open at all times. If this is too much, just hug the pillow and rest the upper body, bending as far forwards as you can.

## Benefits

The Standing Forward Bend stretches the back of the legs, detoxifying the entire body, while lengthening and relaxing the whole spine, from the sacrum to the neck. It benefits the digestive and reproductive systems, treats asthma, relieves headaches and corrects hypotension and anemia. It is also recommended as an antidote to spiritual and psychological fatigue.

# Sun Stretches

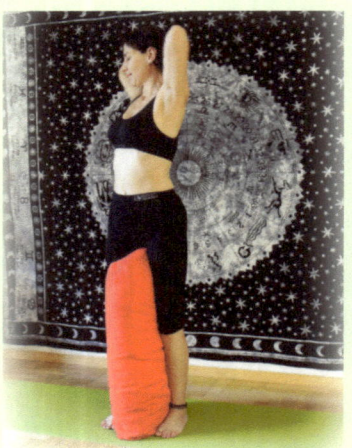
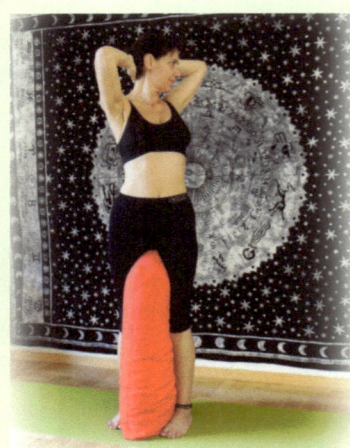

Hold the pillow between the knees, legs straight, grab the floor with the toes and press the feet firmly down on the floor. Support the head with the hands, keeping the elbows open. Inhaling stretch the torso up, exhaling turn to the right. Repeat on the other side. Next inhale, stretch up and exhaling lean the torso sideways, as much as you can. Repeat on the other side.

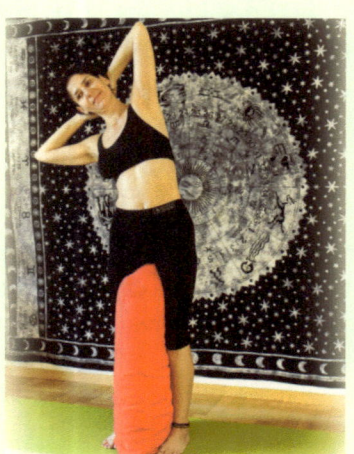
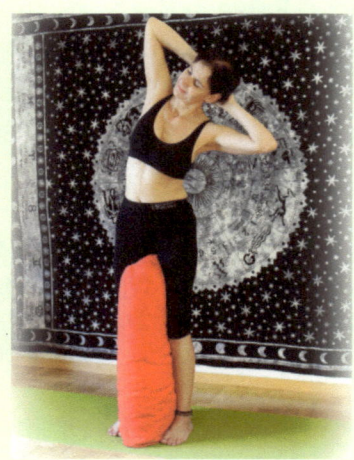

While turning or leaning to the side, always keep the opposite leg strong and the tailbone pointing downwards. This way you secure the right and safe position of the pelvis. If you suffer from scoliosis, stay longer where the shorter side opens. Instead of holding the head, you can stretch the arms up. If you are experiencing arthritis and even lifting the elbows feels difficult for now, just hold your waist with the hands.

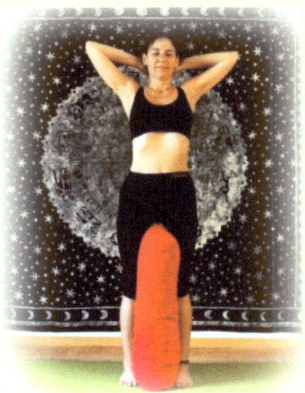

You can also just do a simple stretch up in this position. The pillow helps the legs remain parallel, securing the right alignment of the pelvis.

## Benefits

The Sun Stretches align, lengthen and strengthen the entire body and improve balance and stability. They are therapeutic for problems of the knees and ankles, they correct flat feet, facilitate breathing and calm the emotions and the mind. They are also a very good preparation for standing exercises and an excellent way to start the day.

# Pyramid

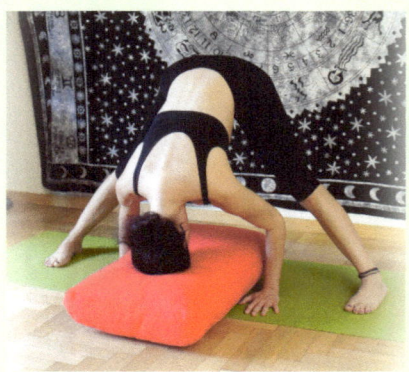

Open the legs wide, hold the feet parallel and grab the floor with the toes, stepping the soles of the feet firmly and evenly. Pull the belly in, extend the torso and lean forwards, until the head rests on the pillow. Bring the body weight toward the front of your feet and roll the ankles outwards. Place your hands down and keep a straight back, with the shoulders away from the ears.

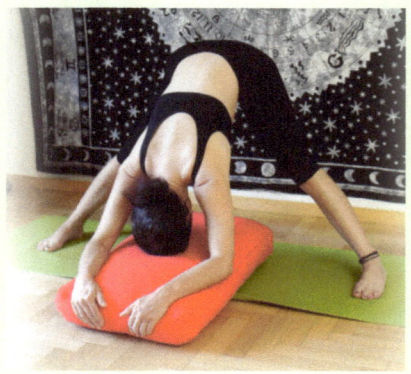

Rest the arms and hands on the pillow, allowing the upper body to relax more. Let the chest sink towards the floor.

If you can't bend that much yet, use two pillows, but remember to touch the head on the tip or the forehead and elongate the neck. Slow exhalations will assist you to folc more. The legs have to be straight and strong. If they get tired, relax them by bending one at a time every now and then. To make it easier, imagine that you are hanging from the ceiling on a strap around your pelvis. This will release some of the tension and you will feel lighter.

To come out of the pose put your hands on the hips and try to lift the back straight up. In case you suffer from back or lower back problems and this feels difficult or painful, just bend the legs in a steady position, curve the back and let the spine unfold slowly and gently, one vertebra after the other, the head last.

## Benefits

The Pyramid strengthens the legs and the back, enhances blood circulation and gives confidence and courage, as the opening of the legs occupies all the space we are entitled to. Also, looking at the world upside down, the mind gets the chance to release old dysfunctional beliefs and open up to new, fresh ideas.

# Great Goddess

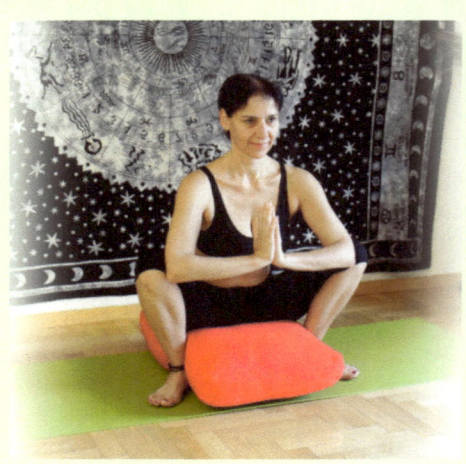

From the Pyramid pose, instead of coming up to a standing position, bring the legs closer, bend them and lower the pelvis until it sits on the pillow. The feet don't have to be parallel anymore, so you can adjust them in a comfortable, steady position. Put your palms together in prayer and push the inside of the knees outward with the elbows to open more, while lengthening the chest and neck upwards. Stay for a few deep breaths. If your heels don't touch the floor, open the legs more. Also you can put the hands down for support, until you become familiar with the pose and your hips can open wide enough.

This is the natural position for giving birth. Women had brought their babies into the world for thousands of years this way, using the spontaneous opening of the pelvis and gravity. It has also been, through the centuries, the resting pose for field workers, who used it to relax their back and legs during their breaks. And the best position to assume when defecating.

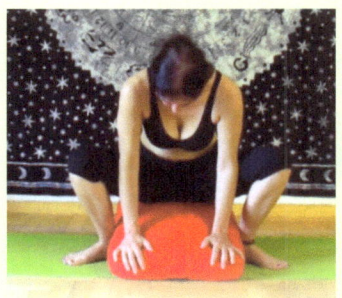

Grab the pillow for support, if sitting down fully feels difficult for now. Hold the legs strong and steady while you are adjusting the pelvic floor.

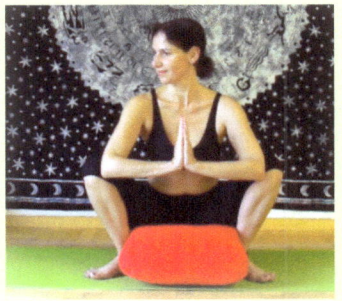

You can gently turn the head left and right, to free the neck from any tension. This will help the spine elongate more.

## Benefits

The Great Goddess position strengthens the legs and relaxes them from the tension caused by prolonged standing. It helps treat constipation and colitis. It lengthens the spine and greatly benefits the reproductive organs. An excellent hip opener, especially useful for the last month of pregnancy, because it leads to easy childbirth.

# Upward Facing Dog

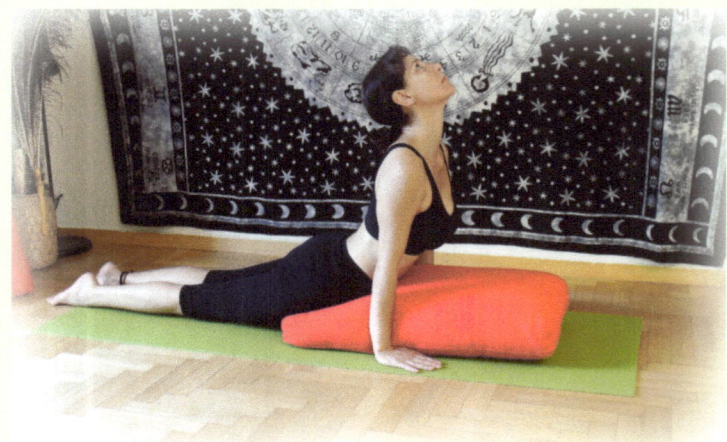

Place the palms next to the sides of the rib cage. On the inhalation lift the trunk. Hold the elbows parallel, stretch your arms and legs at the same time, lifting the knees slightly off the floor. Keep your feet together and active by pushing the foot bridges down. Open the chest, lengthen and look upwards, while pressing the palms firmly and evenly onto the ground.

## Benefits

The Upward Facing Dog strengthens the back, arms and buttocks, lengthens and rejuvenates the spine. Benefits the digestive system, increases appetite and gives a glow to the skin by detoxifying the kidneys. It can treat scoliosis, stiffness of the hips and rounded back problems, while strengthening and lengthening the legs. It gives the benefits of aerobic exercise to the heart, stimulates blood circulation, relieves fatigue and depression and regulates the thyroid. The pillow softens the effort required for the full posture and prepares the body for it.

# Sphinx

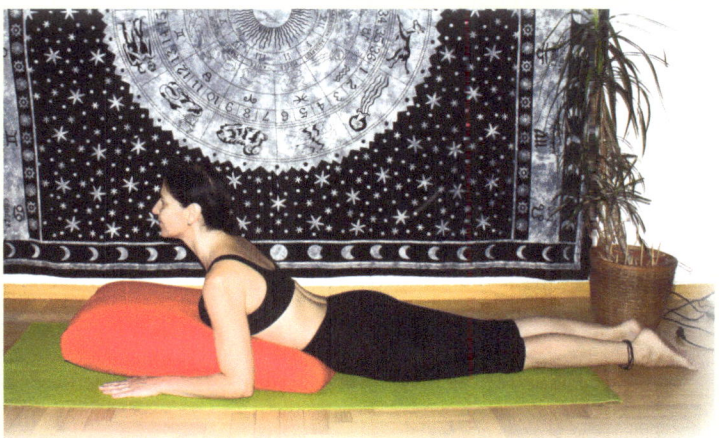

Lie with the pelvis on the floor and the chest on the pillow. Bring the elbows and hands parallel. Open the shoulders and lengthen the neck, looking straight ahead. Keep the legs together and active. Hold still and steady. It's a pretty easy posture to stay for a few breaths and an excellent preparation for the Upward Facing Dog.

## Benefits

The Sphinx gives all the benefits of the Upward Facing Dog in a milder form. Regular practice will eventually lead you to the more difficult pose, where you can enjoy its benefits to the fullest. It is a very good pose to cultivate motionlessness, stability and patience.

# Locust

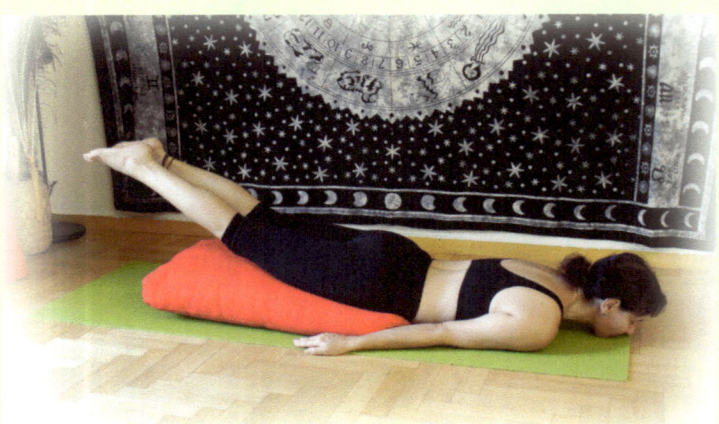

Lay on your stomach, with the pelvis on the pillow, the chin on the floor and the hands beside the body, palms facing down. With the inhalation lift the legs. Keep them strong and together, in order to add stability and protect the lower back. If lifting both legs is too much for now, try to lift one at a time.

Come out of the pose carefully, by relaxing the legs and placing the palms next to the chest and push them down to lift up safely and come to a kneeling position.

## Benefits

The Locust strengthens the back and buttocks, lengthens and rejuvenates the spine, energizes the digestive system and increases appetite. It improves the functioning of all the abdominal organs and corrects scoliosis, stiffness of the hips and rounded back problems. It also stimulates blood circulation throughout the whole body.

# Snake

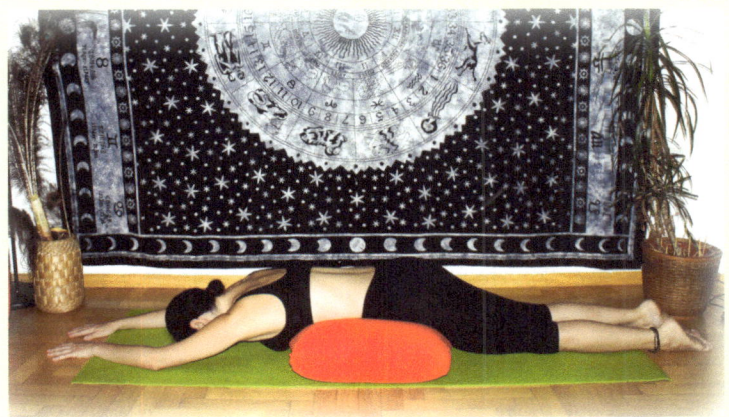

Place the long side of the pillow under the stomach and just relax on it. Extend the arms forward, let the forehead rest on the mat and loosen up the legs. Just breathe and let go with every exhalation.

If you feel that your back and lower back need more rest and alignment, kneel in the Embryo pose, place the pillow on the legs and lean on it.

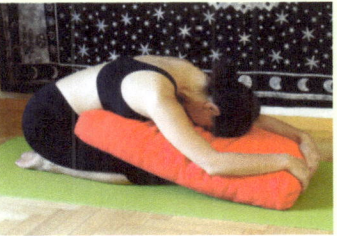

## Benefits

The Snake on the pillow is a counter pose to the Sphinx, Upward Dog and Locust. It relaxes the spine and legs after the stretch and gives the heart a rest.

# Pose of the West

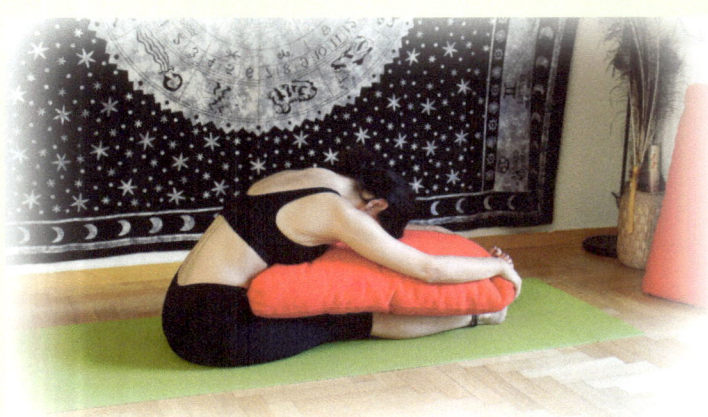

Sit with the pelvis steady on the floor and extend the legs to the front. Place the pillow on the thighs, touching the belly, even pushing it in a little. Straighten your legs, if you can, or at least keep them together with both knees looking up. Take a deep inhalation and lengthen the torso. Exhaling bend forwards as much as you can. Hug the pillow and let the forehead rest on it.

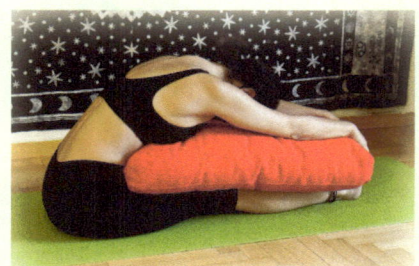

If you are up for more stretching, straighten the arms, bring the elbows closer and grab the pillow from the front. Let the chest sink more and keep the neck long and the shoulders back.

It is called the pose of the West, because the body closes down and adjusts to the end of the day, when the physical functions calm down and prepare for the night.

It stretches the back and legs and relaxes the shoulders, benefits the liver and kidneys and improves the function of the digestive and reproductive systems. It relieves insomnia, hypertension and sinusitis, reduces obesity, calms the mind and facilitates communication with the inner self.

According to the ancient yoga scripts, it is the best among the postures, as it stimulates the breathing and digestive channels and frees the body from diseases.

······························ Tip ··························

You can also sit on a pillow, to make it more comfortable.

To help the treatment of scoliosis, stretch the short side more.

In case of lordosis, place your hands under and pull the buttocks slightly back before you start bending.

For kyphosis, turn the thigh muscles slightly inwards.

Avoid exercise during pregnancy and the first days of menstruation, also if you are experiencing a lower back ache crisis.

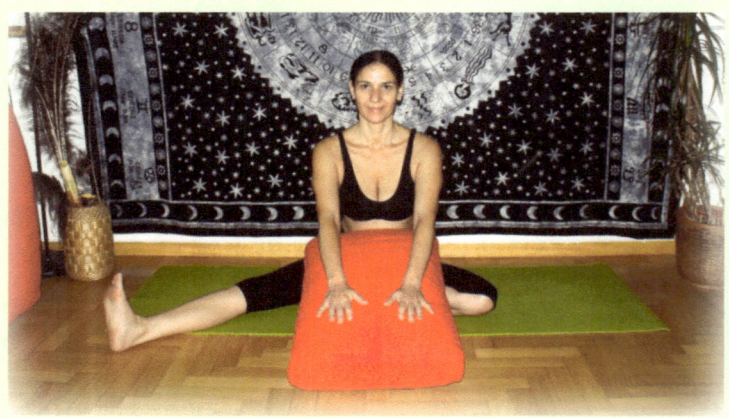

Extend one leg to the side. Fold the other and place the heel of the foot on the inner thigh of the extended leg, touching the perineum. Put the pillow on top and adjust it to your belly. Lift the torso and open the chest.

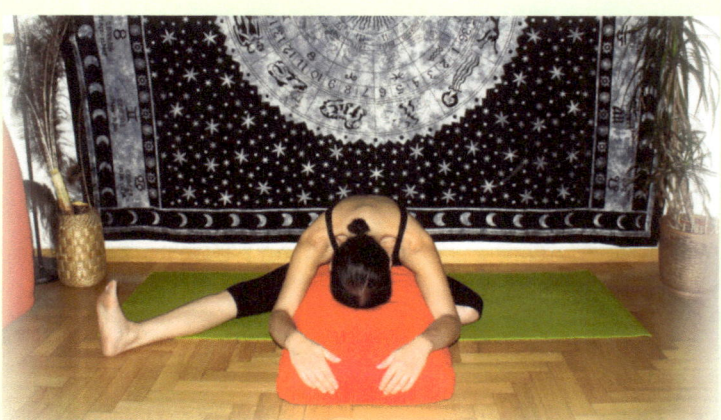

Extend forwards and hug the pillow. Breathe, pulling the belly in with each exhalation. Elongate and straighten the

You can sit on a folded blanket to give the tail bone more comfort. Practice very carefully if you are suffering from a back injury or chronic back pain. To help the extended eg stretch more, you can point and flex the toes or gently roll the ankle outwards a few times.

upper body as much as possible. Hold your pelvis firmly and evenly on the floor at all times. Keep the extended leg strong, knee and toes pointing up.

If you are struggling, use two pillows one on top of the other to make it easier. If, for any reason, you cannot bend forwards at all yet, just sit and keep stretching your spine. With practice you will eventually fold all the way.

Repeat with the other leg and hold the pose for the same amount of breaths.

## Benefits

It strengthens the back muscles, stretches the spine and shoulders and treats scoliosis. It also stimulates the liver and kidneys and improves digestion. It increases fertility, relieves the symptoms of menopause, fatigue, headache, menstrual discomfort, high blood pressure, anxiety and insomnia. It calms the brain and treats mild depression.

# Seated Wide Angle

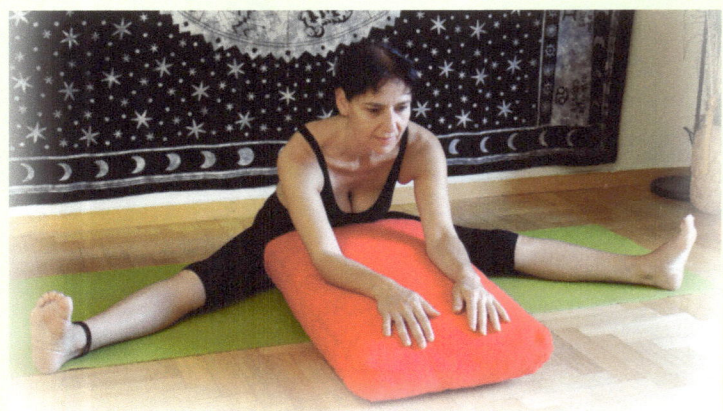

Open the legs, so that the pelvis sits steadily and evenly on the floor. Place the pillow in between, lengthen the torso and start extending forwards, using the exhalations to stretch further.

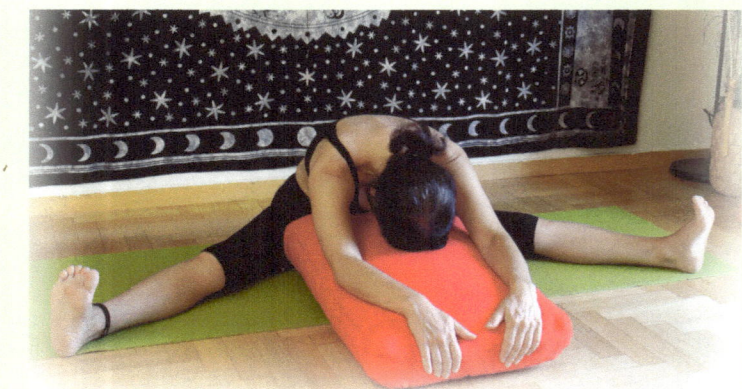

If you can go all the way, hug the pillow and rest the forehead. Straighten the legs and breathe, relaxing in the position, thus allowing the body to open more.

You can use a folded blanket as a support for the tail bone. Take it easy or avoid if you are suffering from a back injury or chronic back pain.

Open your legs only to the extent that it feels comfortable, not exceeding your limits. To secure the right position for the pelvis, turn the thigh muscles slightly inwards with your hands. This way the upper body has a good basis to stretch and expand, otherwise it will tend to curve and lean back.

If it's too difficult, use two pillows. And if bending forwards is, for any reason, impossible for the moment, just stay with the legs open and elongate the torso, energizing the abdominal and back muscles. Keep the legs strong and active, with knees and toes facing up.

## Benefits

The Seated Wide Angle calms the brain, stretches the insides of the legs and loosens up the hip bones. It also strengthens the spine, stimulates the abdominal organs like the liver, the intestines and the kidneys, releases sexual energy and regulates the menstrual cycle. An ideal exercise for late pregnancy.

# Butterfly

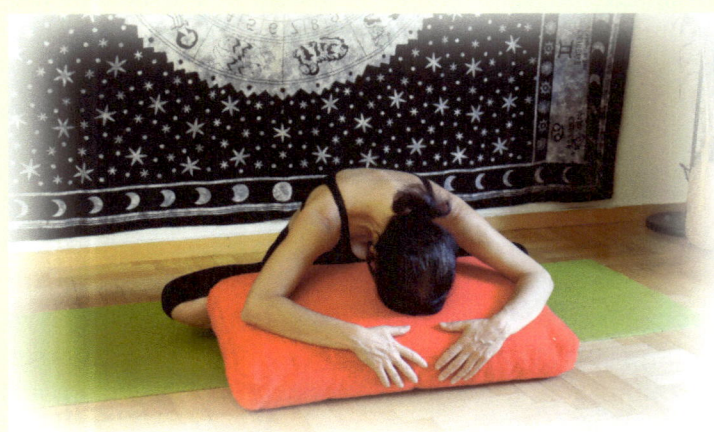

After the Seated Wide Angle, the Butterfly pose is necessary to relax the legs from the intense stretch. Put the soles of the feet together and place the pillow on top. Let your trunk lean forward. The more you lean, the more the legs open to the side. Breathe deeply and evenly and use the exhalation to relax the inner thigh muscles. The legs must feel as light as a butterfly's feathers.

## Benefits

The Butterfly relaxes the legs, pelvis and back. It benefits the digestive and reproductive systems and frequent practice during pregnancy facilitates childbirth. It calms the mind and, according to the ancient yoga scriptures, destroys all diseases.

The Supine Butterfly, while maintaining all the benefits of the seated position, also opens the chest, making breathing easier. It can be utilized as a relaxation pose, instead of the one in p.64.

# Supine Butterfly

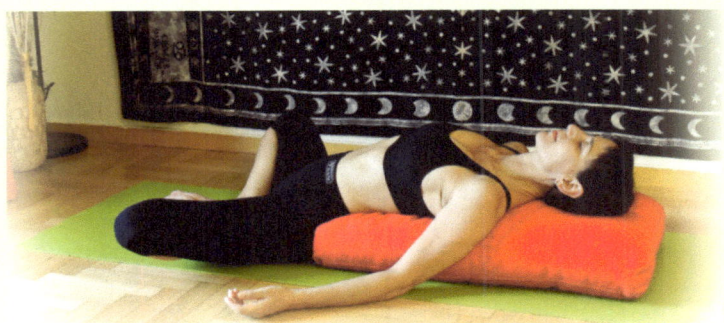

Put the soles of the feet together and place the pillow behind your buttocks, centered to the tailbone. Using your hands for support, lean back gradually and carefully, spread the spine evenly on the pillow and finally let the head rest. Open the arms on the sides, loosen up completely and stay as long as you like. This position is ideal for deep, full breathing. To come up safely, bring the knees together and turn on one side, until your back is off the pillow.

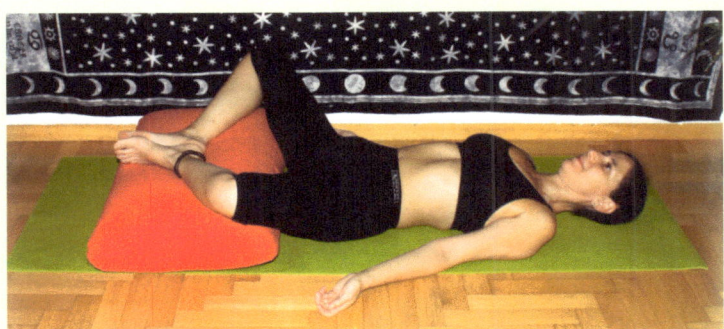

Another version is to lie on your back and rest the legs on the pillow, soles of the feet together. Very effective for relieving tired legs after standing or walking for too long.

# Plough

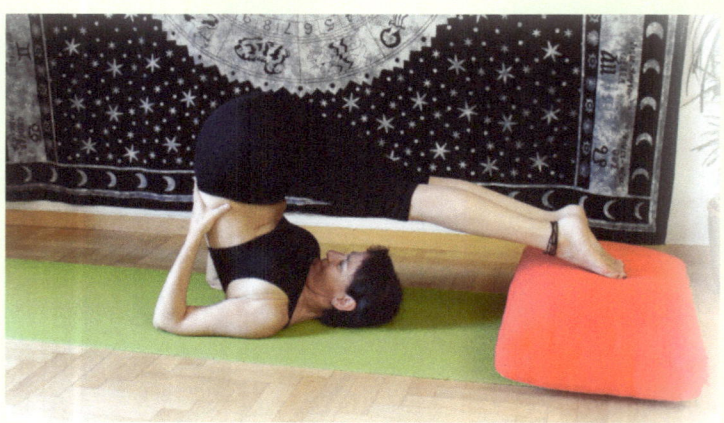

Lie on your back and place the pillow behind the head, approximately the distance of another same size pillow. After a few attempts you will find the exact right distance, according to your height. Bend the knees, push up and lift the pelvis. Support the back with the hands and activate the abdominals. Now bring the feet one by one or both together behind the head and let the toes touch the pillow. If they don't, you may need two pillows one on top of the other or you can just bend the knees and rest them on the forehead. If they do, you can add movement by walking the knees without lifting the toes. Stay for a few breaths and push the coccyx towards the head as much as possible, respecting the limits of your lower back and neck.

To come back, put the palms down and slowly let one vertebra at a time return to the floor. Keep your legs strong and together and the abdominals active. When the entire spine is safely down and the pelvis fully spread on the mat, you can continue lowering the legs slowly, to exercise the abdominals more.

If your neck feels stiff, put a folded blanket underneath and don't stay too long in the position. If the problem is severe, avoid it completely. Definitely avoid during the first days of menstruation and late pregnancy.

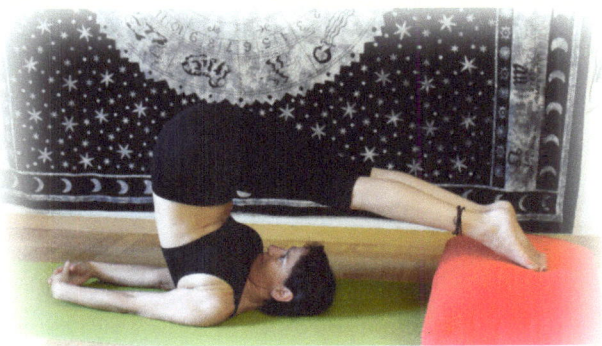

If you are comfortable with the toes touching the pillow, interlace the fingers and stretch your arms away from the shoulders, making space for the neck to lengthen. You can bend and straighten the legs, until you get used to the position and prepare for the final, where the toes touch the floor directly.

## Benefits

The Plough lengthens the entire back of the body, relaxes the heart, cleans the lungs, improves eyesight and hearing and maintains healthy gums and teeth. It prevents and cures colds, skin aging and wrinkles. It activates the digestive and reproductive systems, regulates the thyroid and blood pressure and burns belly fat. It stimulates the nervous system and contributes to the treatment of multiple sclerosis. It calms the mind by relieving stress, headaches and insomnia.

# Fish

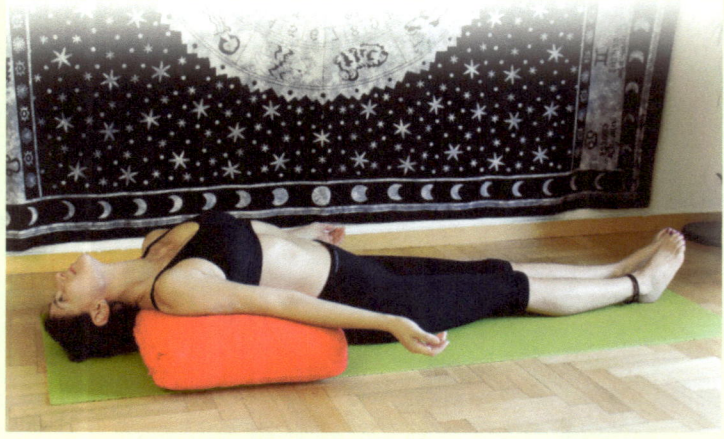

The Fish is the counter pose for the Plow and it is necessary to be performed after it. Place the long side of the pillow behind the buttocks and carefully lean back, spreading your spine on the pillow. Relax the neck, touch the top of the head on the floor and keep the legs straight, together and active. Don't move the head left or right. Breathe deeply and evenly.

Keep opening the chest, while the pelvis remains steady and heavy on the floor. Look up towards your forehead, to give the eyeballs a good therapeutic massage.

If the neck feels uncomfortable, come up, place a folded blanket in that spot on the mat and try again.

To release the pose bring the head back first and push the hands on the floor to help the torso come up safely to a seated position.

If you are experiencing neck problems, don't stay too long in the position or avoid it completely. Also avoid during the first days of menstruation and late pregnancy.

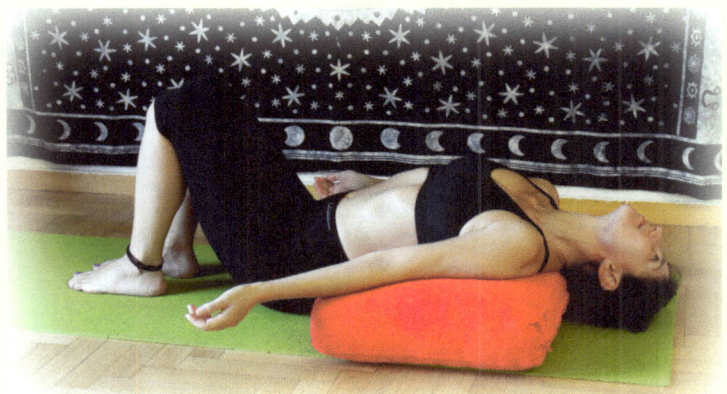

You can also bend your legs, as long as the soles of the feet step steadily and evenly and the knees remain parallel. To sit up from this pose, powerfully grab the outer thighs for support.

## Benefits

The Fish relaxes the neck, corrects the arch of the back and removes the tension from the shoulders. It lengthens the front of the leg muscles and relieves sciatica. It regulates the thyroid, increasing metabolism. It cures sinusitis, improves smelling capacity, facilitates breathing and can stop the nighttime teeth grinding. It gives flexibility to the spine, stretches the abdominal organs and relaxes the mind.

# Waterfall

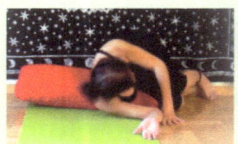

Place the pillow parallel to the wall and lie on it on the side, pushing the buttocks against the wall. Turn on your back, lift your legs and spread the spine evenly and comfortably on the pillow, letting the head and shoulders on the floor. If it doesn't feel right, rather come down and go up again until the pose feels comfortable.

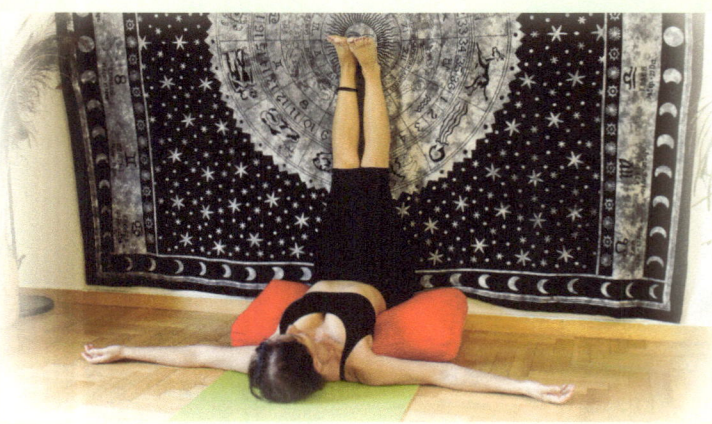

Softly extend the legs, just enough to keep the heels on the wall and the knees parallel. Open your arms to the sides and relax. You can let your head gently turn from side to side, to release tension in the neck. Look up to the ceiling or close your eyes. Stay as long as you feel like and breathe. To come back, bend the knees and turn to the side.

While you are lying on your back you can open the legs. Attempt to keep them as straight as possible and respect your limits. Every exhalation helps the inner thigh muscles relax and open more. You can also extend the arms behind, giving the spine a good stretch.

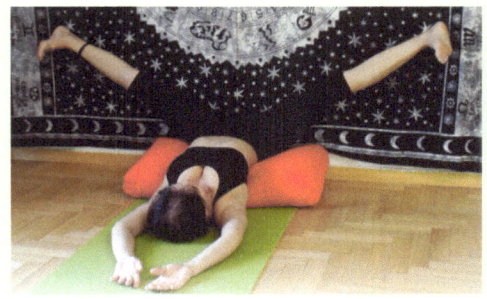
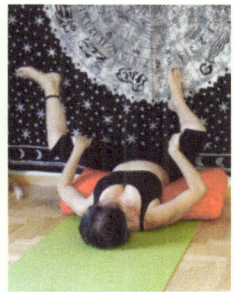

Help the legs close with your hands, as they will probably feel a bit numb and sensitive after such an intense stretch.

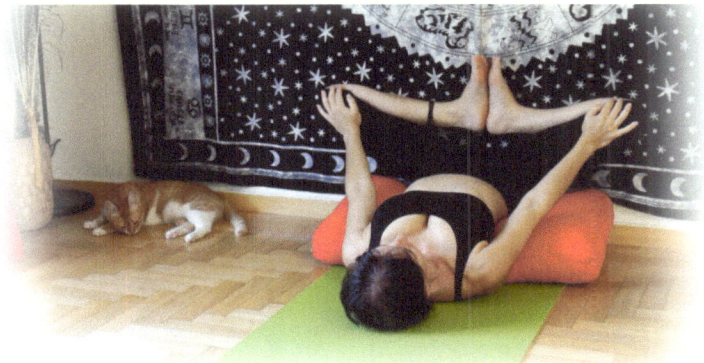

Put the soles together, in an inclined Butterfly pose. Gently press the inner thighs with the hands, opening the pelvic area as much as possible. The cat is optional.

## Benefits

The Waterfall straightens the back, relaxes the body, treats varicose veins, headaches and insomnia. Benefits the digestive and reproductive systems and facilitates breathing. It calms the mind and relieves depression. Like all inverted poses, it rejuvenates the body, removes diseases and is considered anti-aging.

# Supine Spinal Twists 1

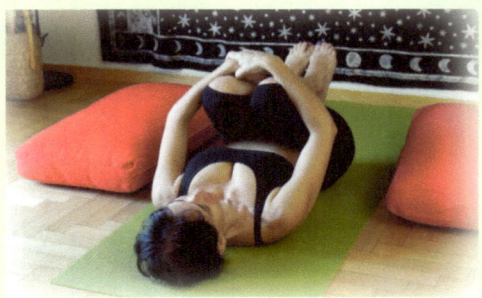

Place a pillow on each side, parallel to the body. Lie on your back and hug the knees onto the chest. Gently rock from side to side, to massage the pelvis and prepare it for the twists.

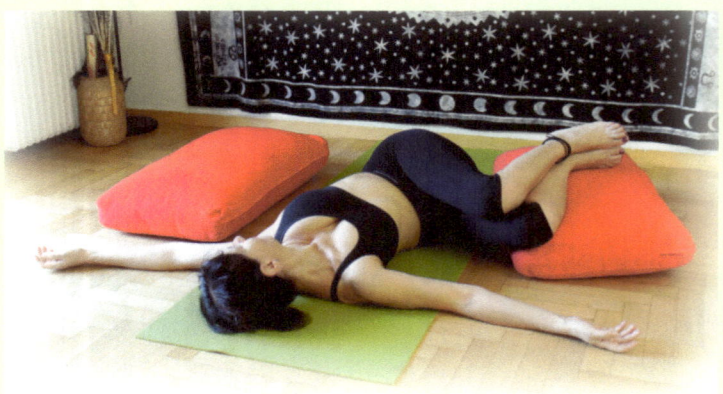

Stretch the arms out, palms up. Inhale and bring the knees closer to the chest. Exhale, turn the knees to the right and let them rest on the pillow. By stretching the left arm more, try keeping both the shoulder blades on the floor. Relax into the pose. With each exhalation pull the belly in, allowing the pelvis and knees to turn more. Let the head gently roll to the other side.

Use gravity and relax into the exhalations for all versions of the Supine Spinal Twists. Also remember to lengthen and open the body in all directions. Arms, neck and torso are stretched and spread generously.

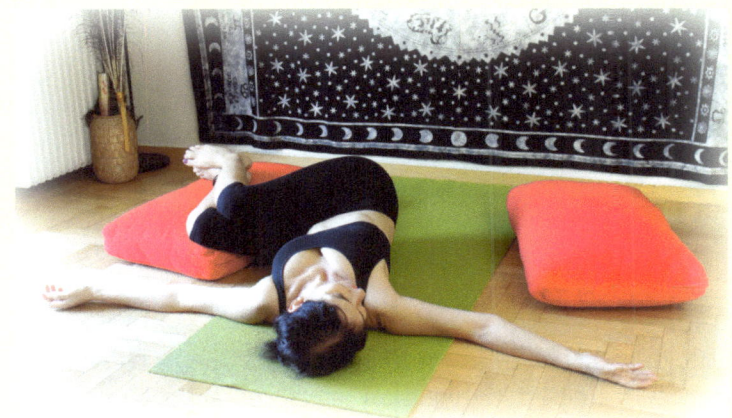

When you feel you have stayed long enough on the right side, inhale and bring the knees back up to the chest. Exhale, let them fall on the left side and repeat the exercise for the same amount of breaths. Finally hug the knees onto the chest again and gently rock the back side to side.

## Benefits

This exercise increases the flexibility of the spine and opens the lungs, facilitating breathing and boosting positive energy. It detoxifies and rejuvenates the abdominal organs, giving health to the entire body and resolves constipation and colitis issues. It burns fat around the belly, preventing and treating obesity and diabetes. It can contribute greatly to the cure of scoliosis if we stretch the short side longer.

# Supine Spinal Twists 2 & Leg Stretch

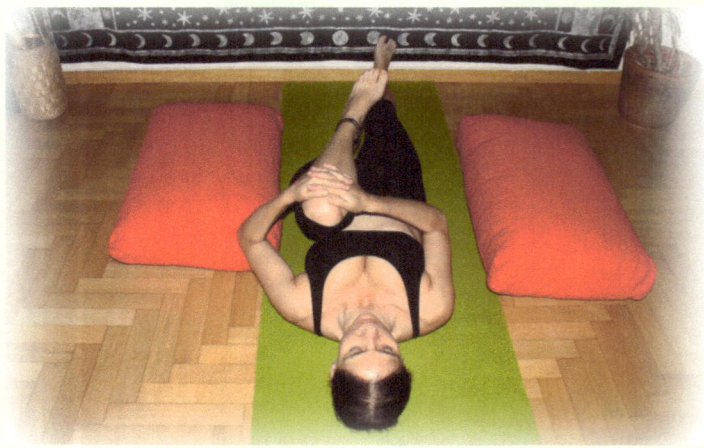

1 Lie on your back between the pillows and hug the left knee close to the chest, while you are stretching the right leg down. For a steady grip, interlace the fingers around the knee. With every exhalation fold the bent leg more, without lifting the shoulder blades or the neck from the floor.

You can also gently roll the ankle outwards and inwards a few times, to treat any stiffness issues and maintain the elasticity of the joint. Keep the extended leg straight, strong and parallel, knee and toes pointing up.

## Benefits

This version of Supine Spinal Twists maintains and increases the benefits of the previous one. The Leg Stretch strengthens and lengthens the legs, aligns the spine and opens the pelvis, benefitting the reproductive organs. It improves digestion, expands the chest, relieves from sciatica and cultivates self-control and peace of mind.

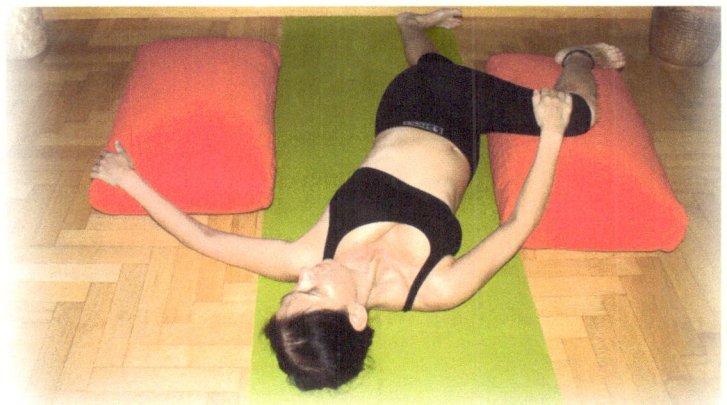

2 Hold the knee on the outside with the opposite hand and push it to the right, until it touches the pillow. Rest the left hand on the other pillow and turn the head towards it. Keep the right leg strong and exhale, pulling the belly in.

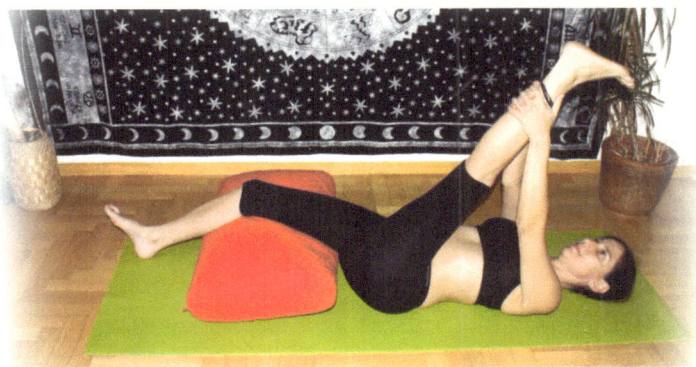

3 Bring back the folded leg and spread your back and pelvis evenly on the floor. After placing a pillow under the right leg, hold the left one either from the calf muscle or the ankle and stretch it, without lifting the shoulder blades or the neck. If it doesn't stretch yet, just keep it bent in a steady position. Repeat all three steps on the other side.

# Upward Extended Feet

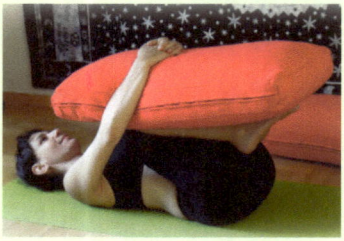 As a preparation, fold the knees, put the pillow on top and hug it. Leave the back side of the body on the floor, from the pelvis to the neck and head and pull the knees closer to the chest.

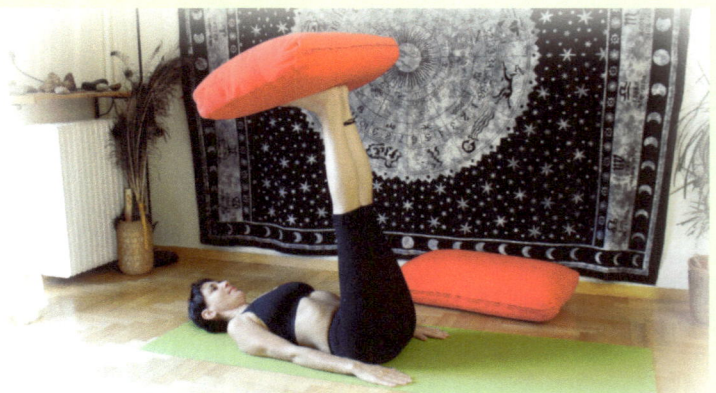

Stretch the legs up, holding the pillow on the soles of the feet. Bend the knees and lift again, keeping the pillow in place. Repeat as many times as you like, using the exhalation to help the lifts. Let the rest of your body flat and relaxed on the floor. Only the abdominals and legs are working. You can press the palms down for support.

## Benefits

It thoroughly exercises the abdominal muscles and stimulates the digestive system, while correcting bad back and lower back posture, removing aches and discomfort. It strengthens the legs and aligns the knees and ankles.

# Resting the Legs

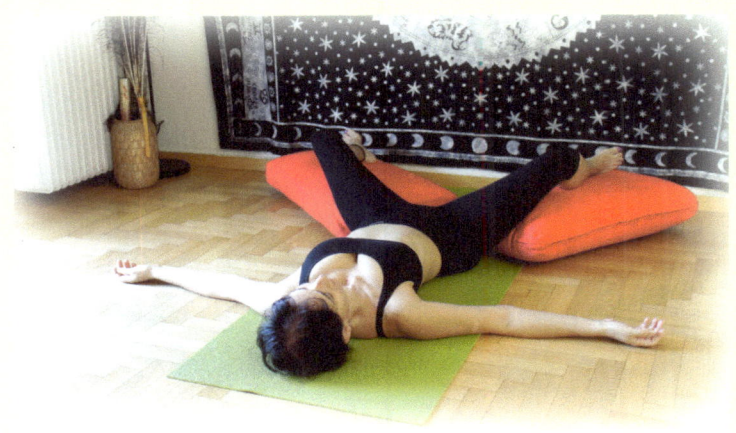

Lie comfortably on your back, open your legs and rest them on the pillows. Make sure your spine and neck are long and straight. Spread the arms on the side, wherever it feels good, and relax completely. There is no effort to be made here at all, it is only a preparation for the final full relaxation and gives almost all its benefits. It could also be the full one for you, if you find it more comfortable than the other.

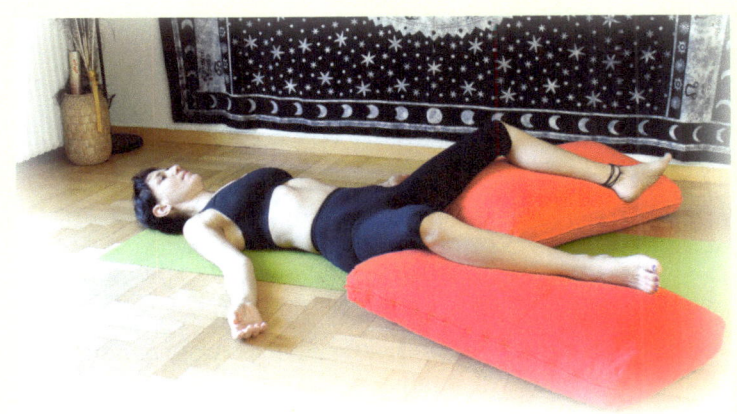

# Bridge

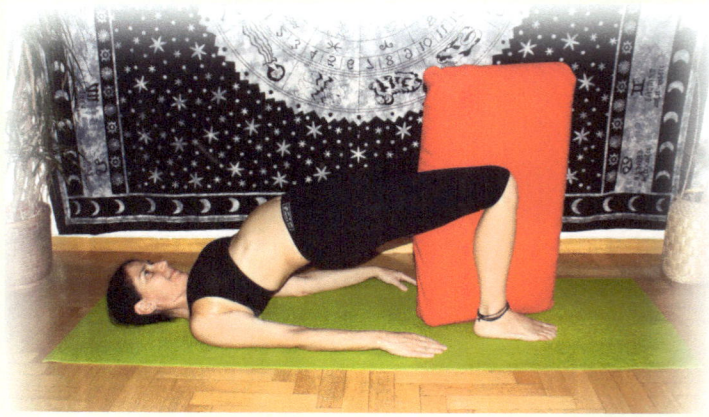

Hold the pillow between your thighs and squeeze it softly, so that your knees stay parallel. Put your arms also parallel on the sides, palms down. Lift the pelvis as high as you can, without dropping the pillow. Hold the head steady and the neck long and relaxed, using the hands for support. The main effort is with the legs and feet. Step evenly and firmly down.

Stay for a few breaths and come down slowly, lowering one vertebra after the other onto the floor. Repeat as many times as you feel up to.

## Benefits

The Bridge strengthens the legs and lengthens the front thigh muscles. It aligns the spine, corrects spinal curvature and facilitates breathing. It relaxes the shoulders and neck, regulates the thyroid function and stimulates the digestive and reproductive systems. It revitalizes the body and relieves depression, mental fatigue, anxiety and insomnia.

# Supported Bridge

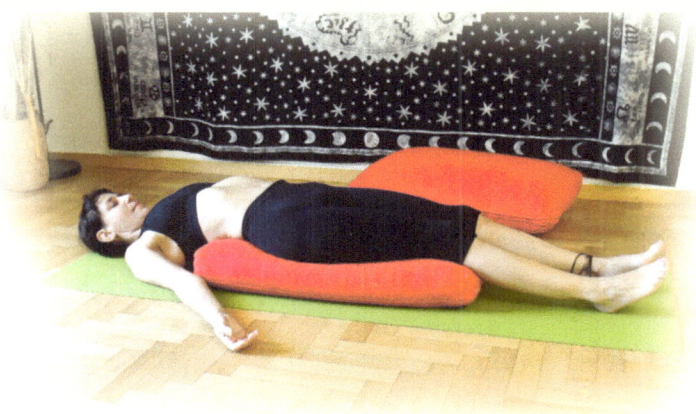

Lie on the pillow with your shoulder blades on the floor. Make sure your spine, including the neck, is long and aligned. Let the arms loose on the sides and relax. You can also use one more pillow under the legs. This is a deeply relaxing pose that aligns the spine, opens the heart and gently stretches the abdominal organs, stimulating digestion. Very effective against stress and depression.

To come up with safety, bend the knees and roll to one side, until you are free from the pillow.

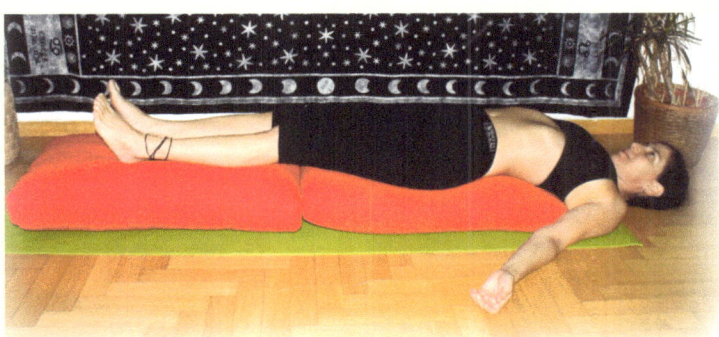

# Relaxation

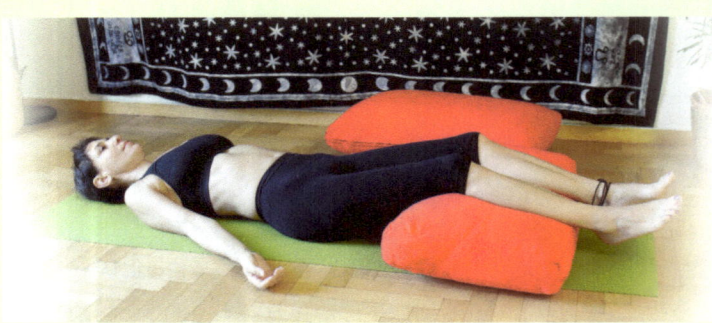

This is the final, deep relaxation. Place a pillow under the knees and lie down, arms by the sides, slightly open, palms up. You can put one more pillow under your back, if you want. Close your eyes and breathe freely. Let every exhalation relax you more. Let thoughts pass through your mind without getting attached to them, like travelling clouds in a blue sky. Imagine the whole body floating or melting. Stay as long as you like. You may want to listen to a guided meditation recording, or you can just follow a relaxing, soothing story in your mind. When you are ready to come up, gently roll on your side and sit up in a steady, comfortable position. Keep the eyes closed for a short while.

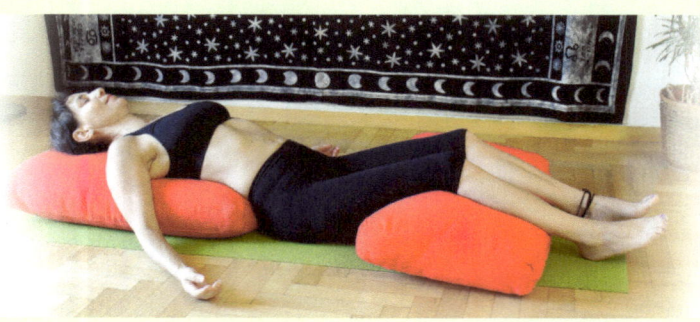

The benefits of deep relaxation are manifold. The blood circulation becomes free and normal, detoxifying the whole body. The muscles relax after the exercise, leaving no stiffness or discomfort. Breathing capacity gets restored and spine blockages released. The heart rests and the cells rejuvenate, wounds heal faster and illnesses are treated. Mental and physical fatigue dissolves. The nervous system and the mind calms down and we enter a state of euphoria. It is always beneficial to practice every day, after exercise or independently.

# Om Chanting

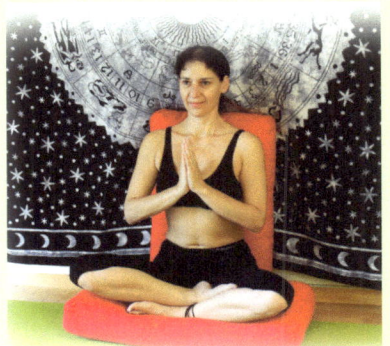

Sit in a comfortable crossed legged position, using the pillows and maybe the wall, too, for support. Join the palms together and chant the ancient sound **Om** three or more times. Feel the vibrations in your spine and internal organs. **Om** is, according to the ancient Hindu scripts, the cosmic sound that created the world and chanting it is therapeutic for the body and mind. It is also a way of expressing gratitude and connecting with Divine Presence. When you are ready, open your eyes.

# Contents

www.ingramcontent.com/pod-product-compliance
Lightning Source LLC
Chambersburg PA
CBHW040323010626
45792CB00024B/2104